DOJO DIET

DOJO DIET

ANONYMOUS NINJA

gatekeeper press
Tampa, Florida

The views and opinions expressed in this book are solely those of the author and do not reflect the views or opinions of Gatekeeper Press. Gatekeeper Press is not to be held responsible for and expressly disclaims responsibility for the content herein.

Dojo Diet

Cover illustration by Debbie Baer

Published by Gatekeeper Press
7853 Gunn Hwy., Suite 209
Tampa, FL 33626
www.GatekeeperPress.com

Copyright © 2023 by Anonymous Ninja

All rights reserved. Neither this book, nor any parts within it may be sold or reproduced in any form or by any electronic or mechanical means, including information storage and retrieval systems, without permission in writing from the author. The only exception is by a reviewer, who may quote short excerpts in a review.

The cover design, interior formatting, typesetting, and editorial work for this book are entirely the product of the author. Gatekeeper Press did not participate in and is not responsible for any aspect of these elements.

ISBN (paperback): 9781662942822

FOR:
FAITH
FAMILY
FITNESS

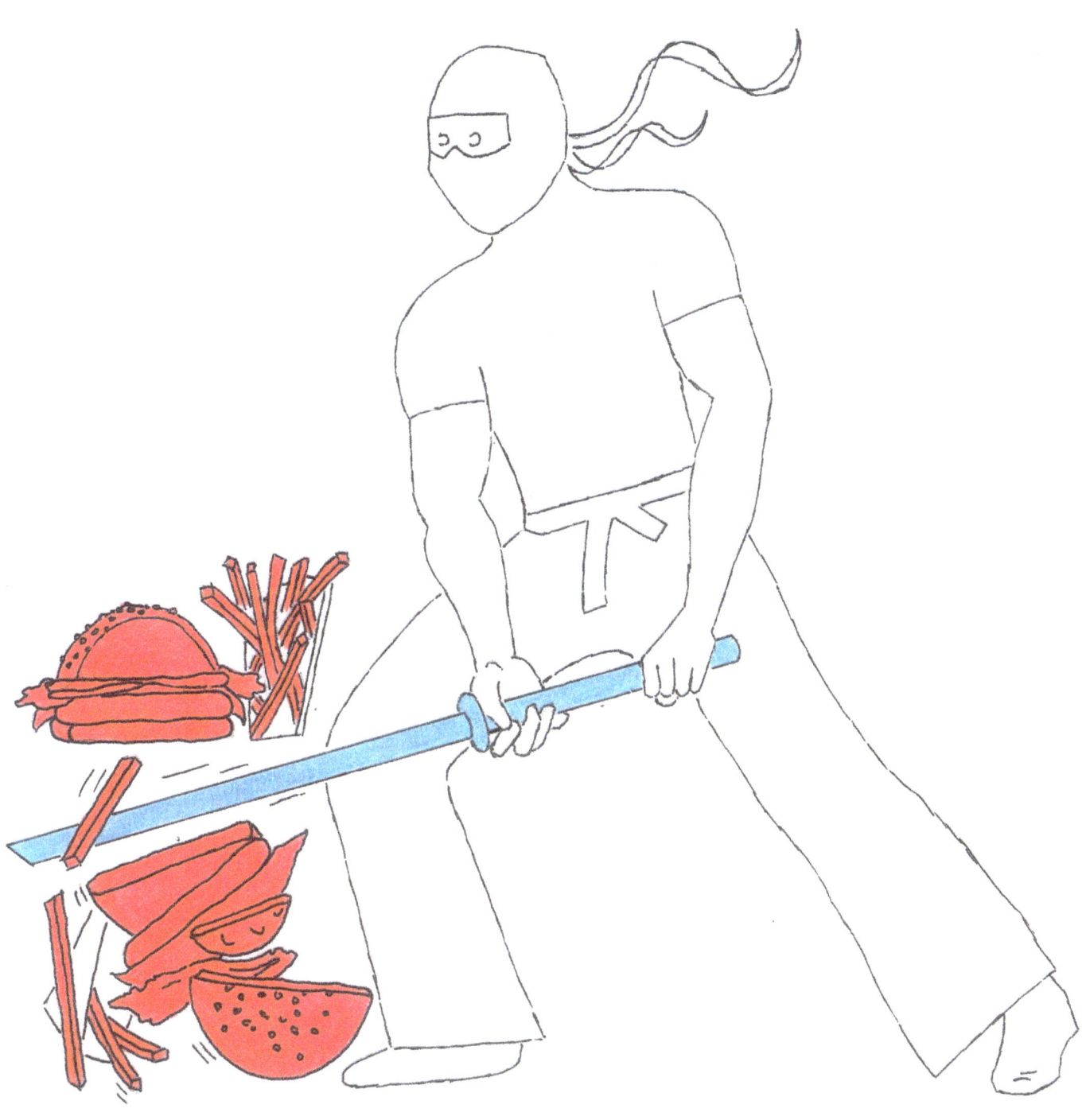

THE DOJO DIET IS A HEALTHY HABIT-BASED LIFESTYLE INSPIRED BY THE NINJA. THE NINJA UNDERSTOOD THE POWER OF HABITS IN CREATING A DISCIPLINED AND BALANCED LIFE.

DID YOU KNOW THAT MOST NINJAS WERE ORDINARY PEOPLE, SUCH AS FARMERS OR MERCHANTS? THEY HAD TO PRACTICE THEIR ARTS THROUGHOUT THE DAY BY COMBINING TRAINING WITH CHORES. IT BECAME THEIR HABITUAL ROUTINE.

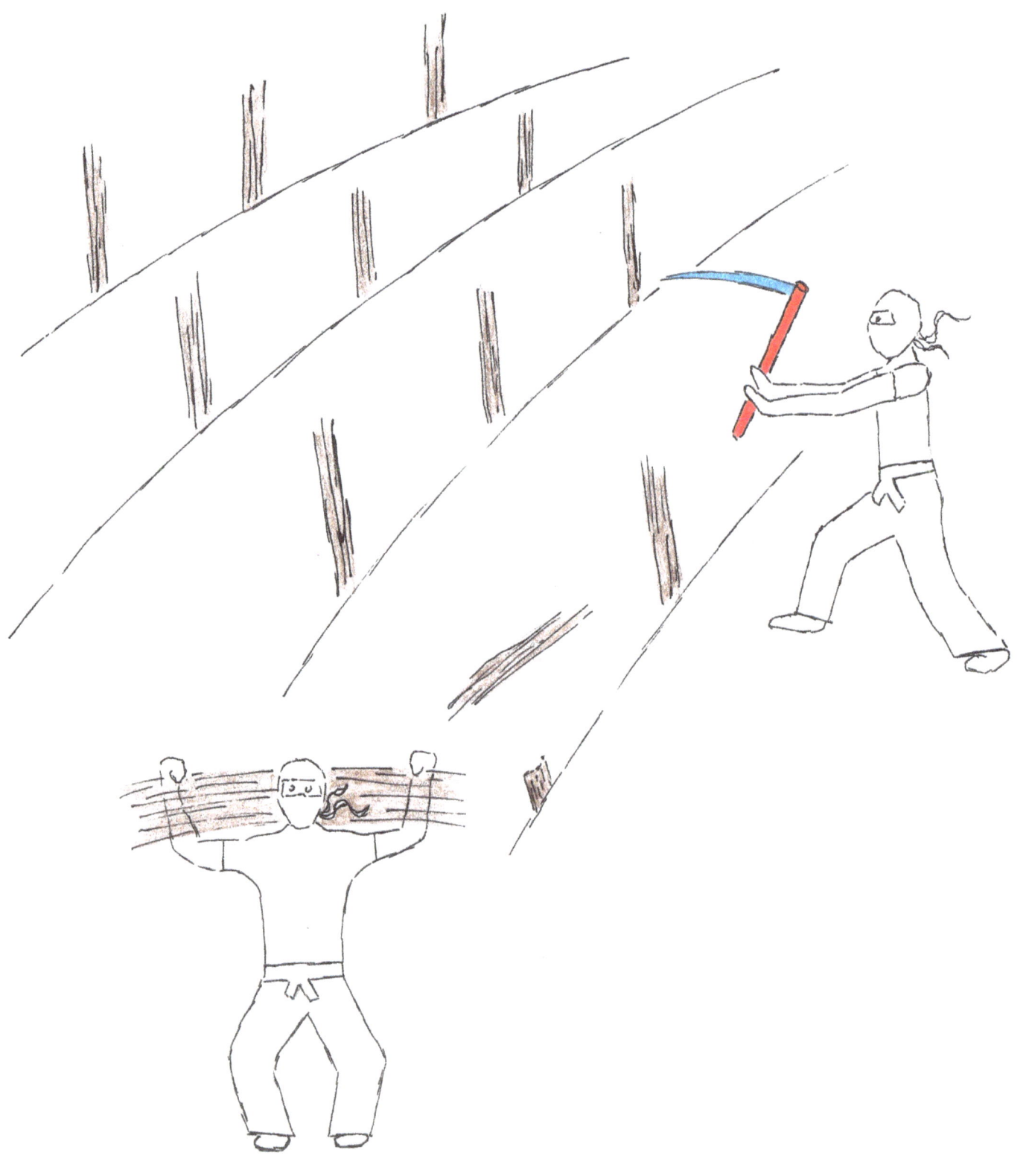

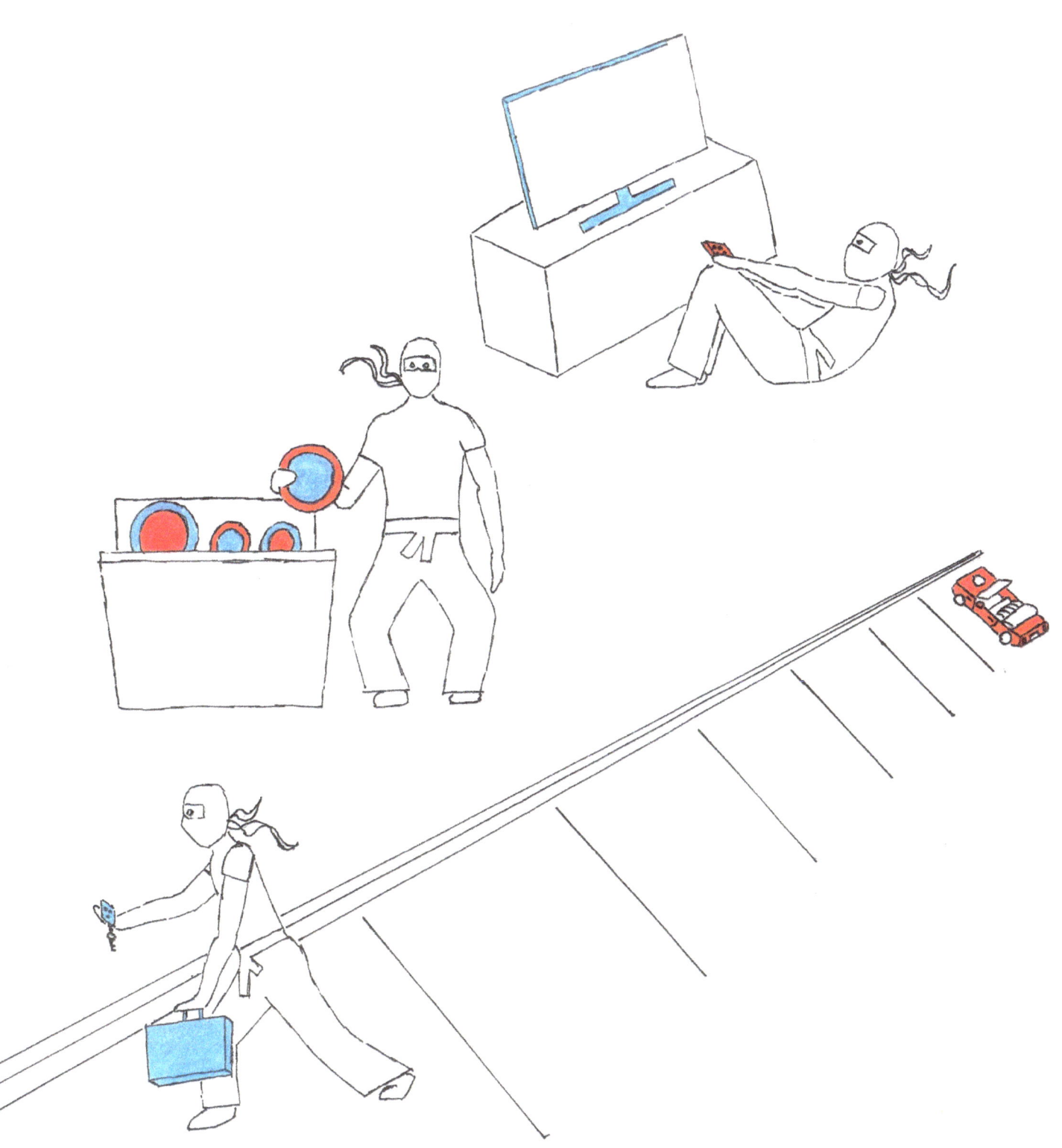

THE DOJO DIET FOLLOWS THE SAME PRINCIPLE OF INCORPORATING EXERCISES INTO YOUR DAILY ROUTINE UNTIL THEY BECOME SUBCONSCIOUS HABITS. IT IS IMPORTANT NOT TO LABEL HABITS AS GOOD OR BAD, BUT RATHER AS CONSCIOUS OR SUBCONSCIOUS, AS WORDS HOLD SIGNIFICANT POWER.

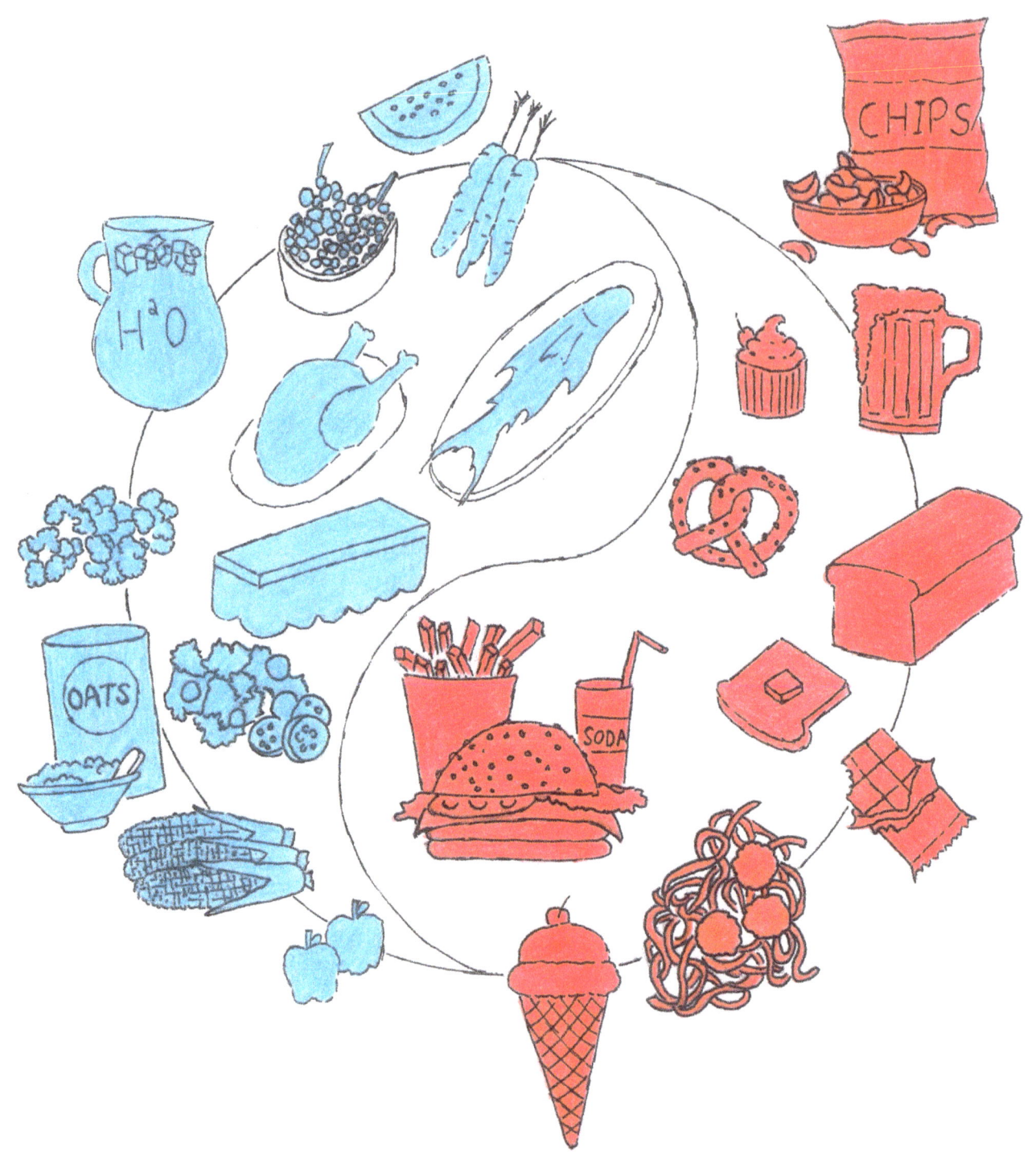

IN ADDITION TO DAILY PHYSICAL HABITS, DIET PLAYS A CRUCIAL ROLE, MUCH LIKE YIN AND YANG TEACHES BALANCE. BY LABELING FOOD AS RED AND BLUE, WE CREATE ACCOUNTABILITY. HOWEVER, IT IS IMPORTANT TO NOTE THAT RED AND BLUE (LIKE HABITS) ARE NEITHER INHERENTLY GOOD NOR BAD. RED REPRESENTS PROCESSED, CALORIE-DENSE FOOD, WHILE BLUE REPRESENTS NATURAL, WHOLE, AND UNPROCESSED FOODS.

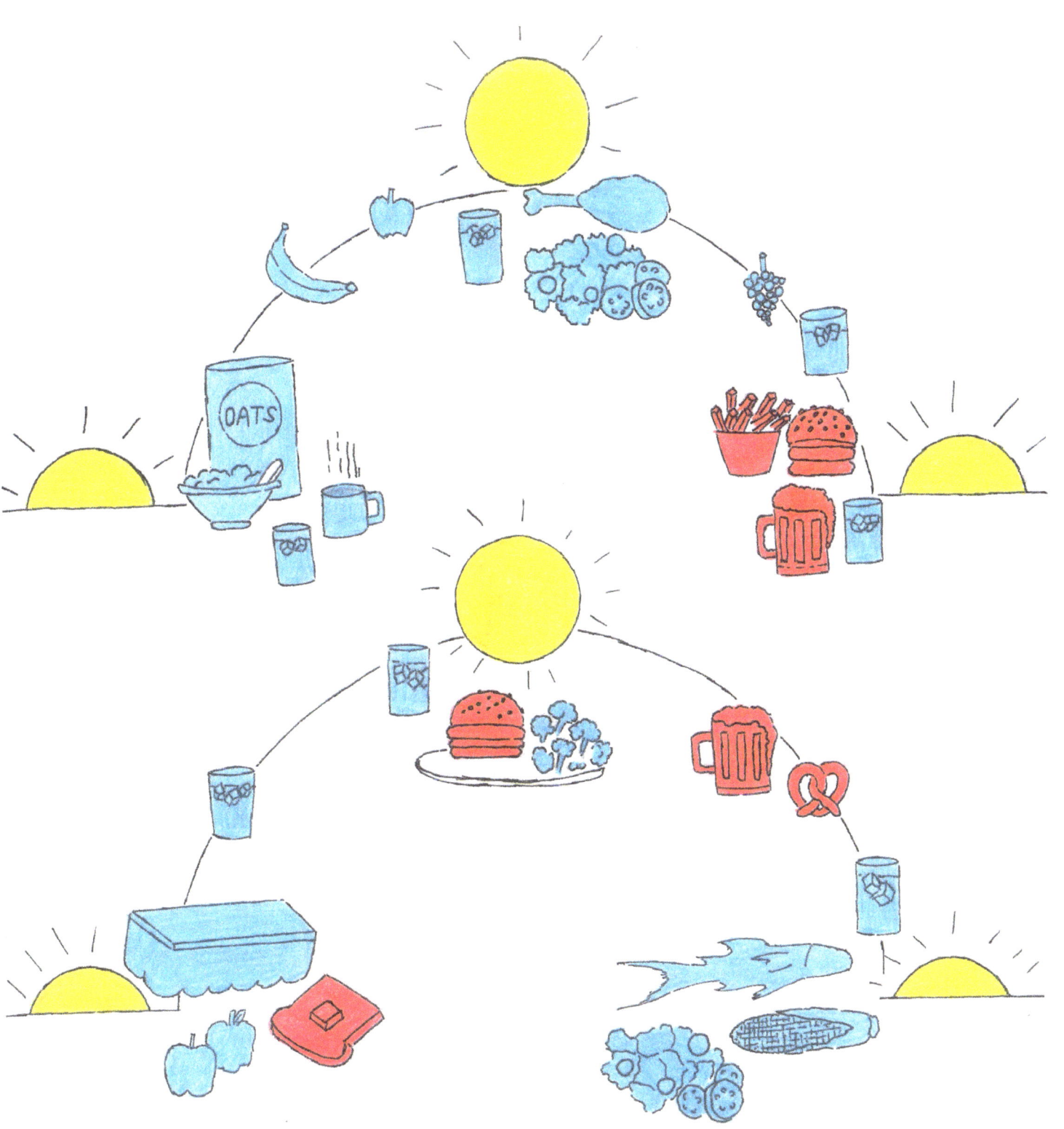

THIS APPROACH HELPS CREATE CONSCIOUS ACCOUNTABILITY FOR YOUR DAILY CALORIE INTAKE AND PORTION SIZES. EACH DAY CAN BE BALANCED BY INCORPORATING A MIX OF RED AND BLUE FOODS INTO EVERY MEAL OR BY HAVING ONE RED MEAL AND TWO BLUE MEALS THROUGHOUT THE DAY.

LET'S DELVE DEEPER INTO UNDERSTANDING THE PHYSICAL HABITS. THERE ARE SEVEN SETS OF SIMPLE EXERCISES, EACH REPRESENTED BY A BELT. BY REPEATEDLY PRACTICING AND EVENTUALLY MEMORIZING EACH GROUP, YOU CAN DEVELOP MUSCLE MEMORY AND ESTABLISH A FUNDAMENTAL HABIT. EACH EXERCISE REPRESENTS ONE OF SEVEN MOVEMENTS (FORWARD, BACK, LEFT SIDE, RIGHT SIDE, TWIST, UP, AND DOWN), PROVIDING A SIMPLE WAY TO INTERNALIZE THE BASIC FUNDAMENTALS. WITH A STRONG FOUNDATION, YOU CAN BUILD A FORMIDABLE EXERCISE ROUTINE, MUCH LIKE CONSTRUCTING A TALL TEMPLE. EACH LEVEL INTRODUCES DIFFERENT COMBINATIONS OR VARIATIONS OF THE FUNDAMENTAL MOVES.

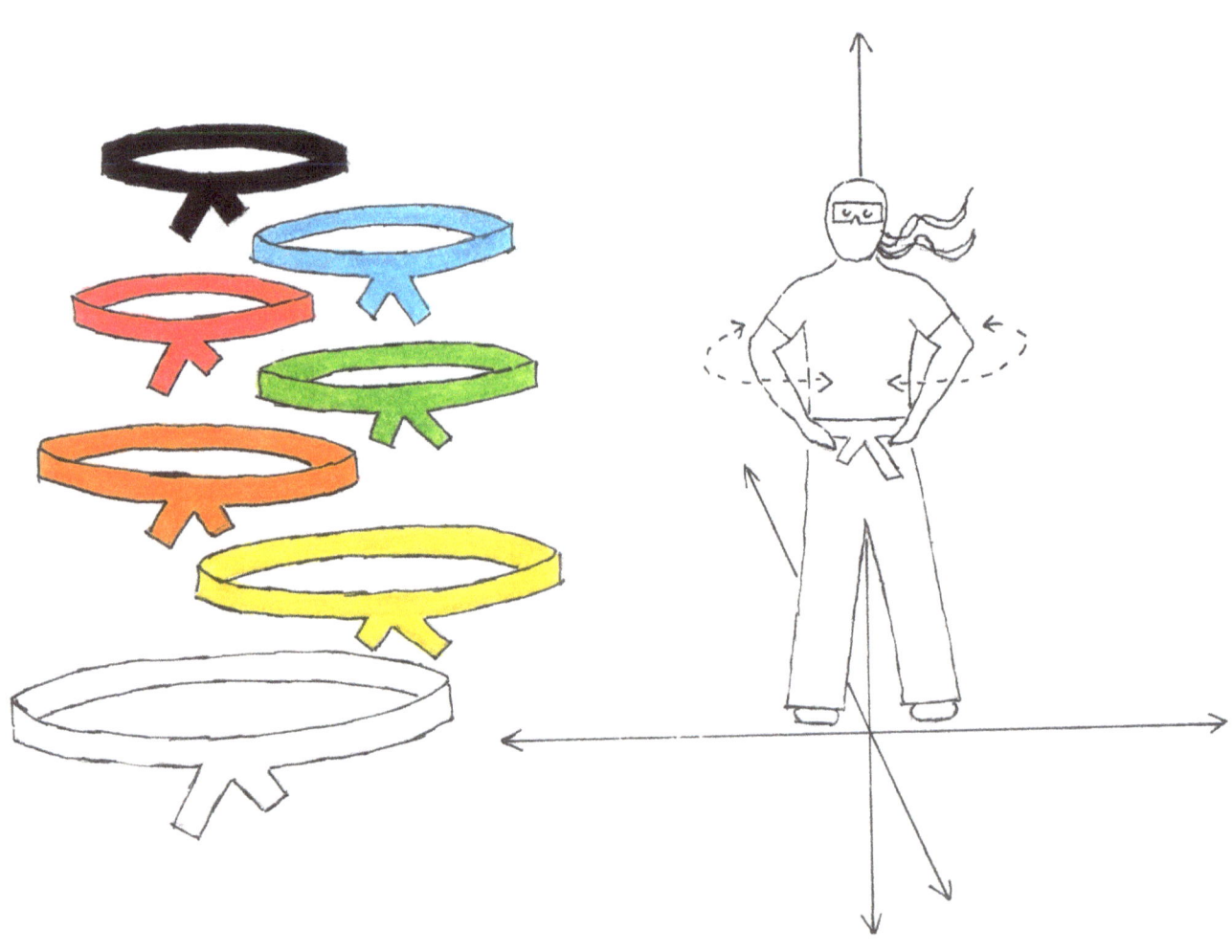

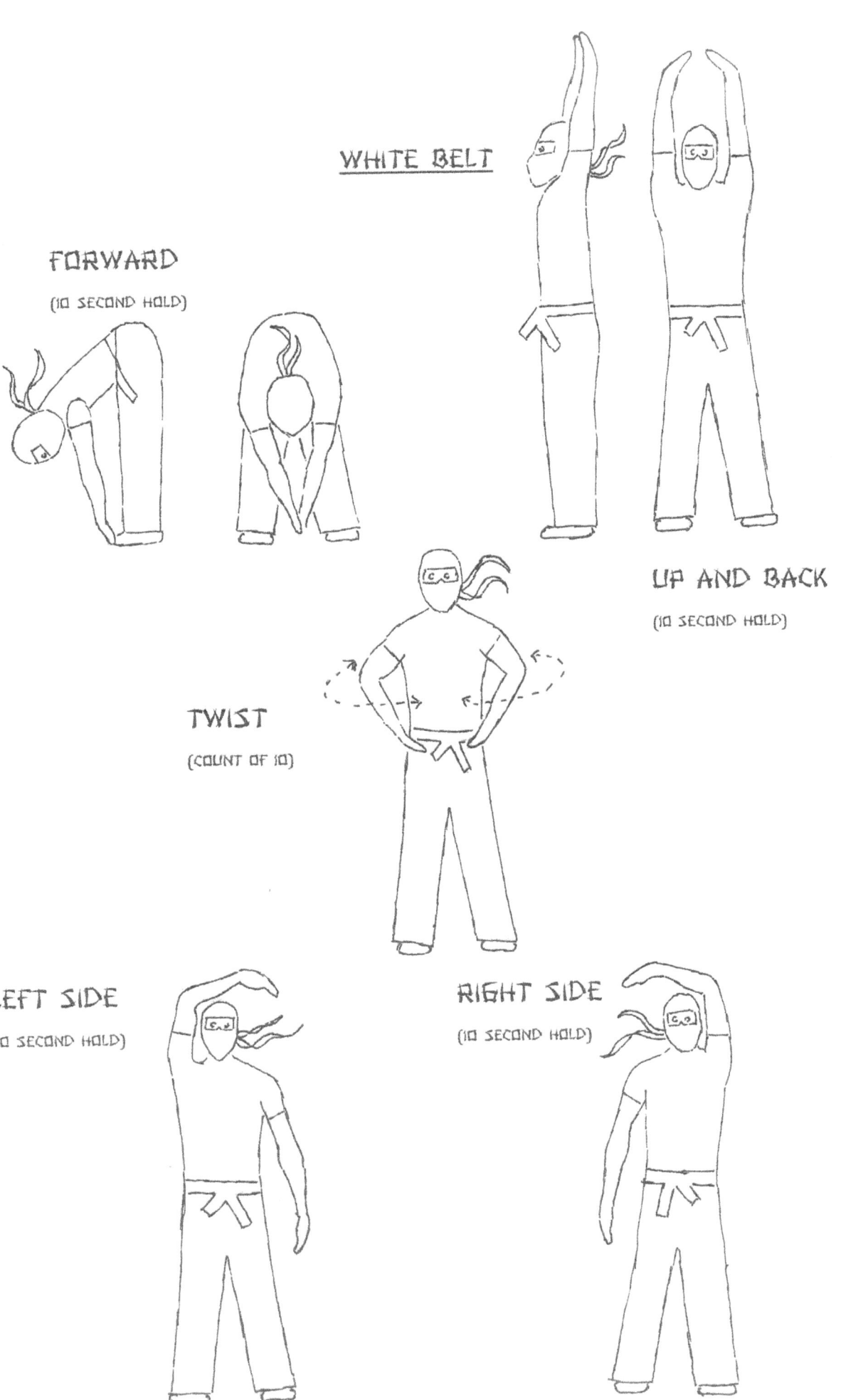

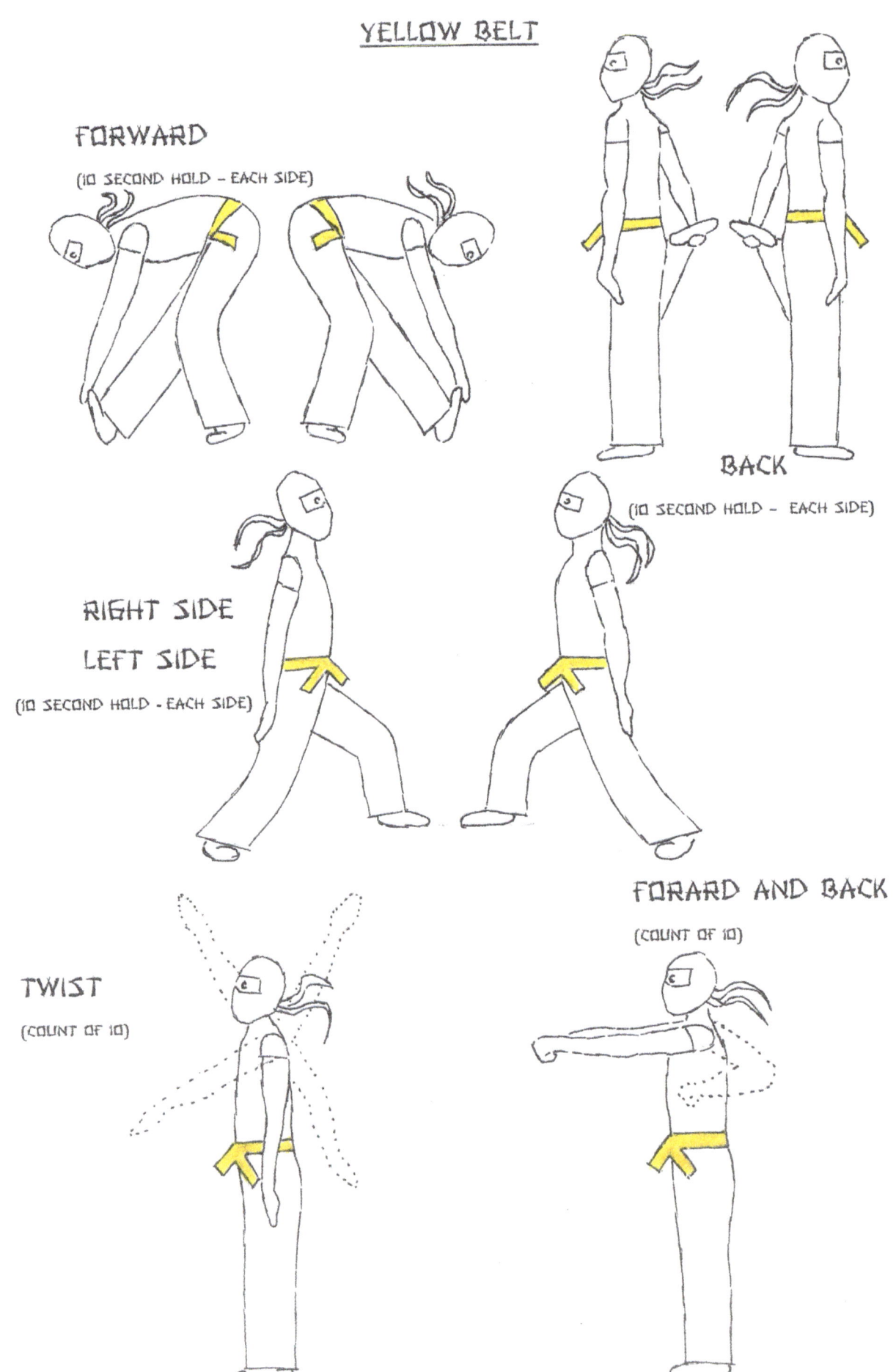

ORANGE BELT

FORWARD (COUNT OF 10)

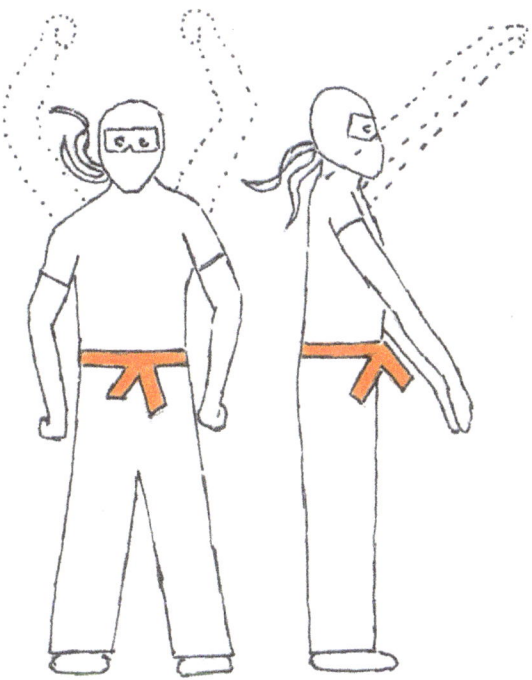

BACK AND UP (COUNT OF 10)

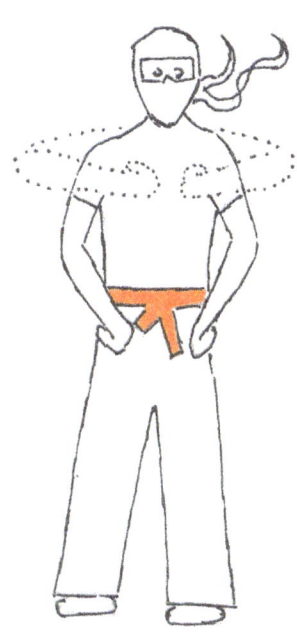

UP (COUNT OF 10)

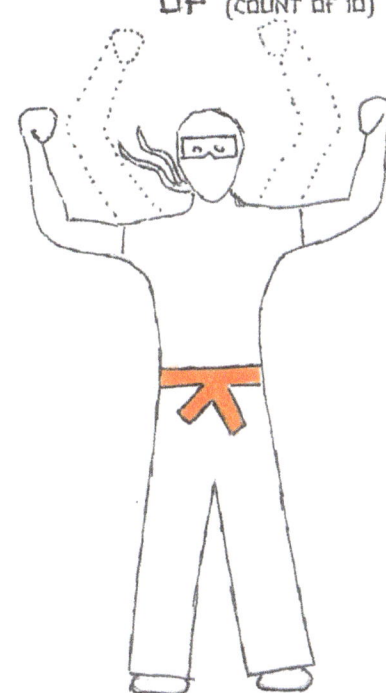

LEFT SIDE RIGHT SIDE (COUNT OF 10)

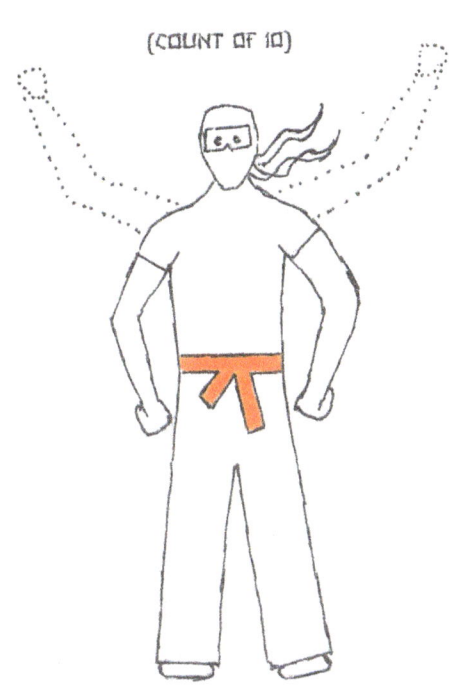

GREEN BELT

FORWARD (COUNT OF 10)

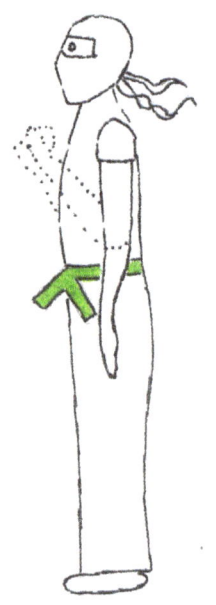

BACK AND UP (COUNT OF 10)

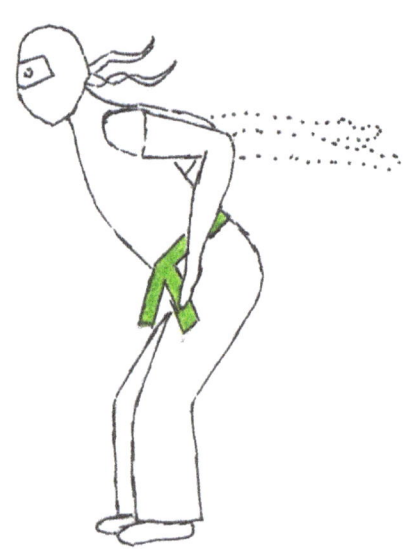

UP (COUNT OF 10)

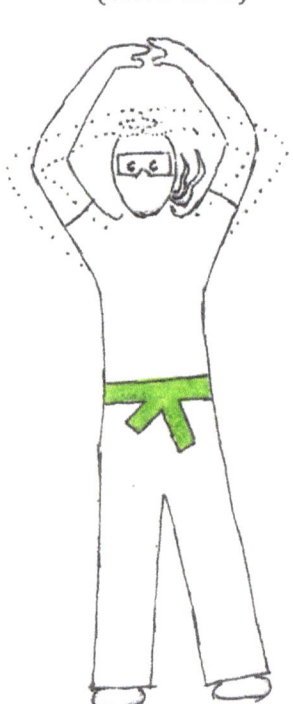

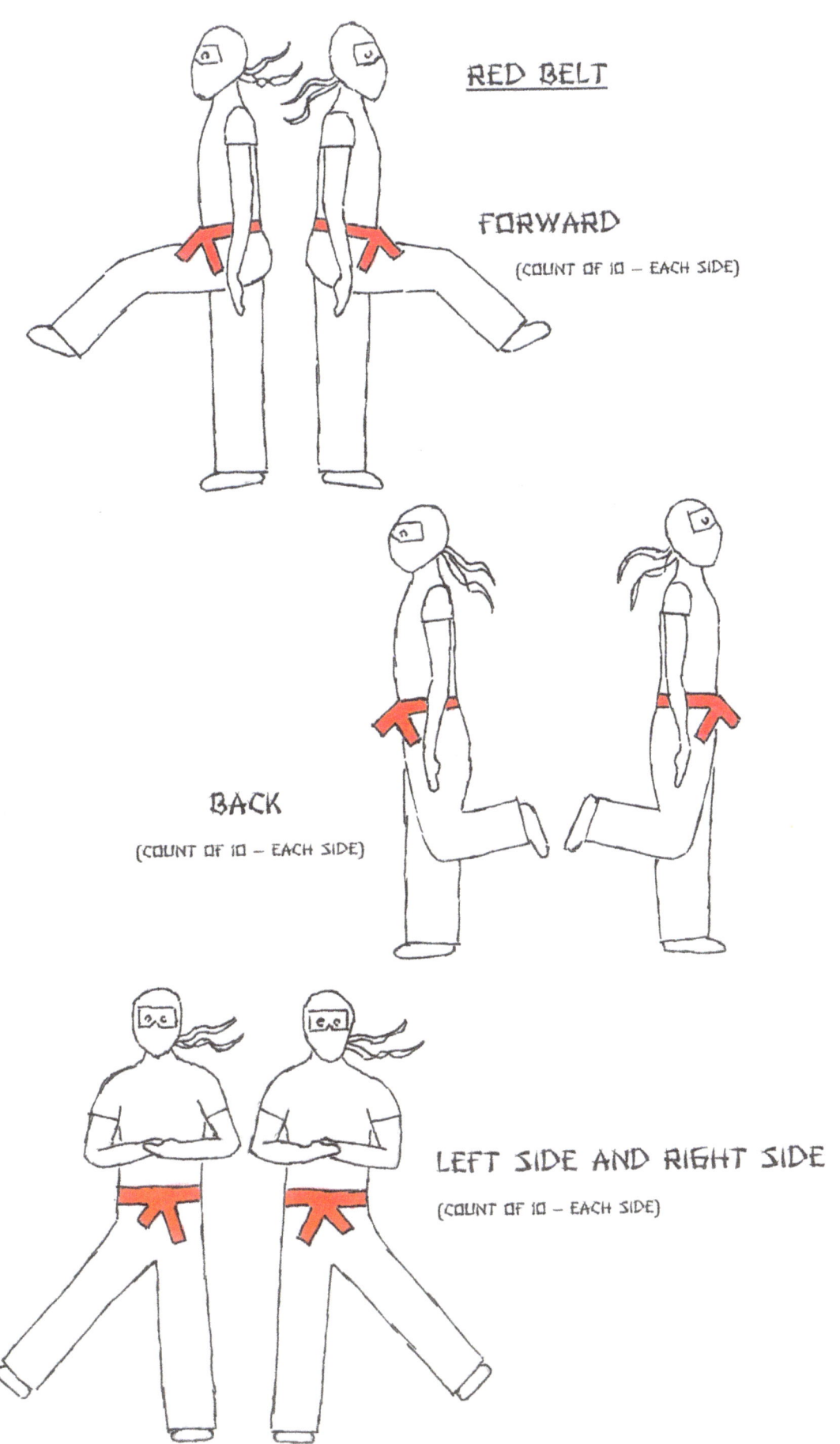

BLUE BELT

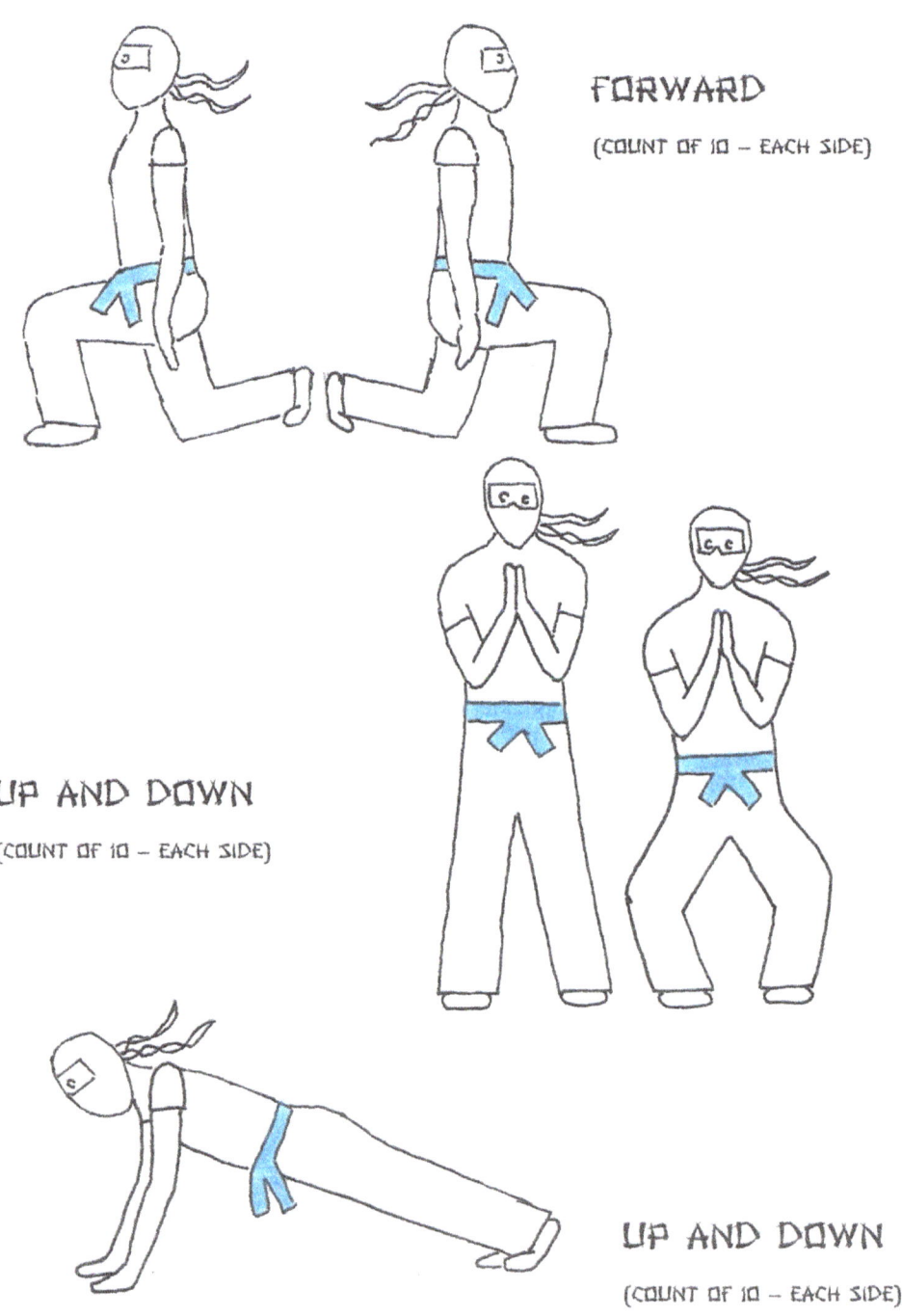

FORWARD
(COUNT OF 10 – EACH SIDE)

UP AND DOWN
(COUNT OF 10 – EACH SIDE)

UP AND DOWN
(COUNT OF 10 – EACH SIDE)

BLACK BELT

FORWARD
(COUNT OF 10)

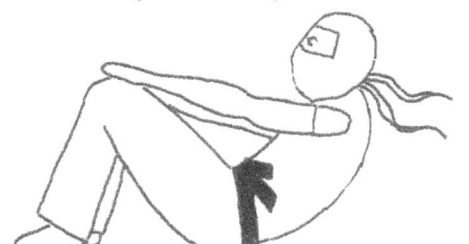

UP AND BACK
(COUNT OF 10)

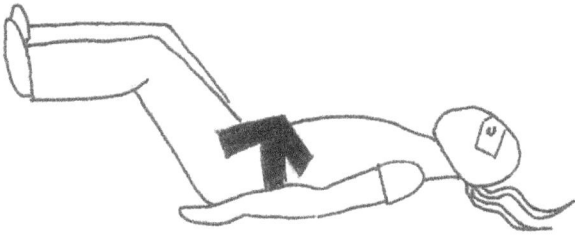

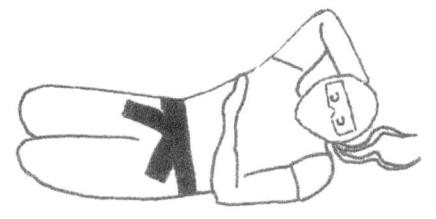

RIGHT SIDE
(COUNT OF 10)

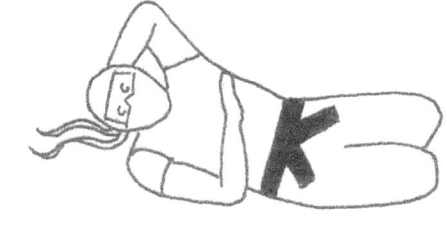

LEFT SIDE
(COUNT OF 10)

WITH THESE SIMPLE IDEAS AND PRINCIPLES, YOU CAN START INCORPORATING MORE MOVEMENT INTO YOUR LIFE AND EXPERIENCE POSITIVE CHANGES. I HOPE THIS DISCUSSION HAS BEEN HELPFUL IN OPENING YOUR MIND TO THE POWER OF HABITS AND HOW THEY CAN CREATE A WELL-BALANCED, WHOLE-BODY FITNESS LIFESTYLE, AKIN TO THAT OF THE NINJA.

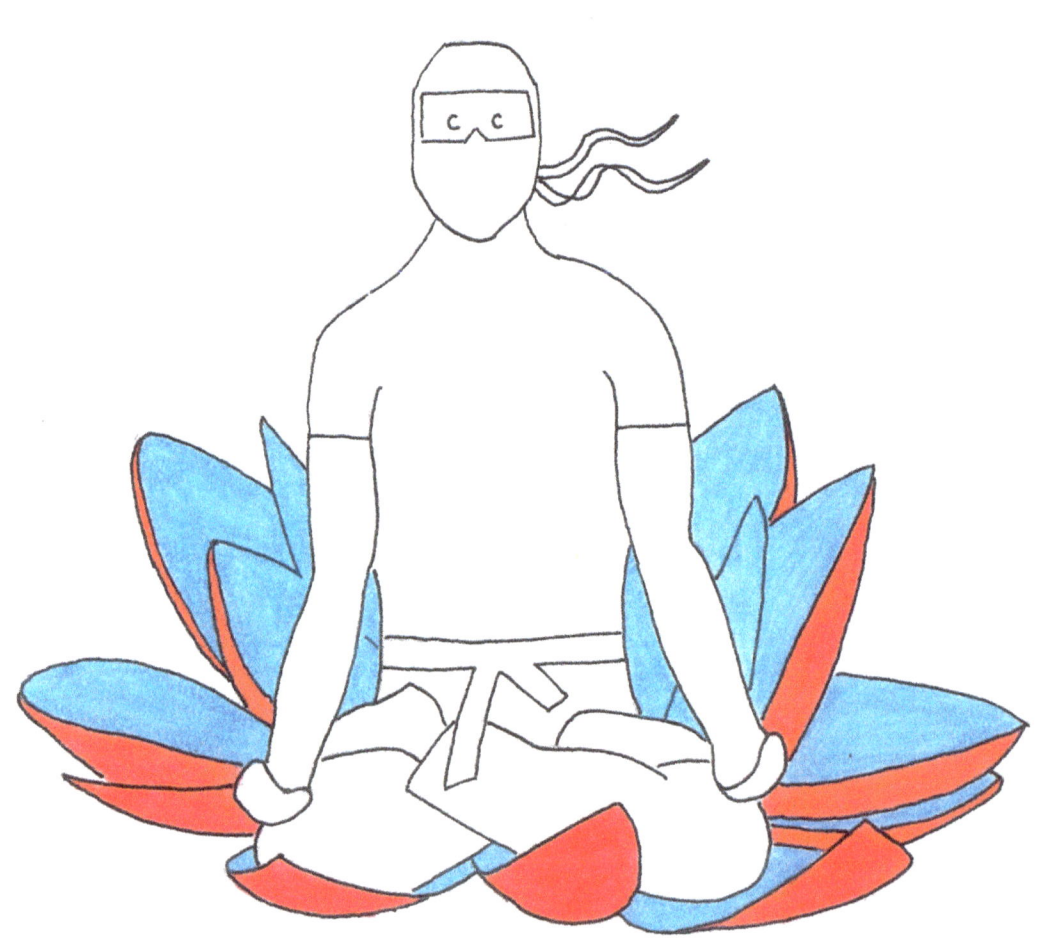